MW01291284

Paleo Cookbook: Ea Stew, Casserole and Skillet Recipes for Busy People on a Budget

by Alissa Noel Grey
Text copyright(c)2016 Alissa Noel Grey

Table of Contents

Delectable Paleo Chicken Recipes for Busy Worknights

The Paleo Diet is one of the best known diets nowadays, probably because it is easy to follow and it achieves great results. You can eat a wide variety of lean meats, healthy fats, vegetables, fruit, nuts and seeds whenever you feel like eating and still lose weight. You never feel deprived and hungry and you never get bored. This is the reason my husband has been following the Paleo diet for the last four months. Naturally I prepare a lot of Paleo meals for him while I still prepare vegetarian meals for the vegetarians in the family. As you can imagine this can be quite time consuming so I am always looking for quick and easy Paleo ideas.

The quick and healthy recipes I am offering in my new cookbook combine fresh ingredients with pantry staples for Paleo chicken meals you can make in minutes. Browse through, pick your fancy and be inspired for cooking Paleo chicken for dinner tonight.

Walnut Pesto Chicken Salad

Serves: 4

Prep time: 10 min

Ingredients:

2 cups cooked chicken, diced

1 large apple, peeled and diced

1 large avocado, peeled and diced

for the walnut pesto

1/2 cup walnuts, chopped

10 fresh basil leaves

1 garlic clove

2-3 green olives

4 tbsps extra virgin olive oil

1 tbsp lemon juice

salt and black pepper, to taste

Directions:

In a food processor, blend together walnuts, olives, basil, olive oil, garlic and lemon juice until completely smooth.

Combine diced chicken, apple, and avocado. Pour over the walnut pesto, stir to combine and serve.

Grilled Chicken Salad

Serves: 4

Prep time: 5 min

Ingredients:

2 cups grilled chicken breasts, diced

1/3 cup black olives, pitted

1 cup grape tomatoes

1 red bell pepper, sliced

3-4 green onions, chopped

1 tbsp balsamic vinegar

1 tsp dried oregano

2 tbsp extra virgin olive oil

salt and black pepper, to taste

Directions:

Place chicken in a deep salad bowl. Add in the grape tomatoes, onion, red pepper and olives. Season with salt and pepper.

Toss gently to combine, sprinkle with oregano, balsamic vinegar and olive oil, and serve.

Chicken and Broccoli Salad

Serves: 4

Prep time: 10 min

Ingredients:

2 cooked chicken breasts, diced

1 small head broccoli, cut into florets

1 cup cherry tomatoes, halved

2 garlic cloves, crushed

1 tsp dried basil

2 tbsp extra virgin olive oil

4 tbsp balsamic vinegar

1/2 tsp salt

Directions:

Heat two tablespoons of olive oil in a non-stick frying pan and gently sauté broccoli for 5-6 minutes until tender. Add in garlic and basil and cook for one minute more.

Place broccoli in a large salad bowl. Stir in the chicken and tomatoes. Season with salt and sprinkle with vinegar and remaining olive oil. Toss to combine and serve.

Vitamin Chicken Salad

Serves: 4

Prep time: 5 min

Ingredients:

3 cooked chicken breasts, shredded

1 yellow bell pepper, thinly sliced

1 red bell pepper, thinly sliced

1 small red onion, thinly sliced

1 small green apple, peeled and thinly sliced

1/2 cup toasted almonds, chopped

3 tbsp lemon juice

2 tbsp extra virgin olive oil

1 tbsp Dijon mustard

salt and pepper, to taste

Directions:

In a deep salad bowl, combine peppers, apple, chicken and almonds.

In a smaller bowl, whisk the mustard, olive oil, lemon juice, salt and pepper. Pour over the salad, toss to combine and serve.

Chicken, Lettuce and Avocado Salad

Serves: 4

Prep time: 5 min

Ingredients:

2 grilled chicken breasts, diced

1 avocado, peeled and diced

5-6 green lettuce leaves, cut in stripes

3-4 green onions, finely chopped

5-6 radishes, sliced

7-8 grape tomatoes, halved

3 tbsp lemon juice

3 tbsp extra virgin olive oil

1 tsp dried mint

salt and black pepper, to taste

Directions:

In a deep salad bowl, combine avocados, lettuce, chicken, onions, radishes and grape tomatoes. Season with mint, salt and pepper to taste.

Sprinkle with lemon juice and olive oil. Toss lightly and serve.

Mashed Avocado and Chicken Salad

Serves: 4

Prep time: 5 min

Ingredients:

2 cooked chicken breasts, diced

1 small red onion, finely chopped

2 ripe avocados, peeled and mashed with a fork

3 tbsp lemon juice

1 tbsp extra virgin olive oil

1 tbsp fresh taragon leaves, finely cut

salt and pepper, to taste

Directions:

Place the chicken in a medium sized salad bowl. In a plate, mash the avocados using either a fork or a potato masher and add them to the chicken.

Add in the onion, taragon, lemon juice and olive oil. Season with salt and black pepper to taste, stir to combine and serve.

Easy Chicken and Egg Salad

Serves: 4

Prep time: 5 min

Ingredients:

2 cups cooked chicken, chopped

2 hard boiled eggs, diced

a bunch of arugula leaves

1 large apple, diced

1/2 cup walnuts, roasted

2 tbsp lemon juice

2 tbsp extra virgin olive oil

salt and pepper, to taste

Directions:

Roast walnuts in a preheated to 450 F oven for 2-3 minutes or until toasted.

In a deep salad bowl, combine chicken, apple, eggs and arugula. In a smaller bowl, whisk lemon juice, olive oil, salt and black pepper. Pour over the chicken mixture. Top with walnuts and serve.

Mediterranean Chicken Soup

Serves: 4

Prep time: 35 min

Ingredients:

3 chicken breasts

1 carrot, chopped

1 small zucchini, peeled and chopped

1 celery rib, chopped

1 small onion, chopped

1 bay leaf

6 cups water

6-7 black olives, pitted and halved

salt and black pepper, to taste

fresh parsley and lemon juice, to serve

Directions:

Place chicken breasts, onion, carrot, celery and bay leaf in a deep soup pot. Add in salt, black pepper and 6 cups of water. Stir well and bring to a boil.

Add zucchini and olives and reduce heat. Simmer for 30 minutes.

Remove chicken from the pot and set aside to cool. Shred it and return it back to the pot. Serve with lemon juice and sprinkled with parsley.

Chicken and Butternut Squash Soup

Serves: 4

Prep time: 35 min

Ingredients:

3 boneless chicken thighs, diced

1/2 onion, chopped

6-7 white mushrooms, chopped

1 small zucchini, peeled and diced

1 cup butternut squash, diced

1 tbsp tomato paste

5 cups water

1/4 tsp cumin

1 tbsp paprika

3 tbsp extra virgin olive oil

Directions:

In a deep soup pot, heat olive oil and gently sauté onion, stirring occasionally. Add chicken and cook for 2-3 minutes. Stir in cumin, paprika and butternut squash.

Dilute the tomato paste in a cup of water and add to the soup. Add in the remaining water and bring to a boil.

Reduce heat and simmer for 10 minutes then add zucchini and mushrooms. Simmer until butternut squash is tender. Season with salt and black pepper to taste.

Paleo Chicken Soup

Serves: 4

Prep time: 35 min

Ingredients:

3 boneless chicken tights, chopped

1 small onion, chopped

3 garlic cloves

1 sweet potato, skinned and diced

1 large carrot, chopped

1 red bell pepper, chopped

1 celery rib, chopped

1 bay leaf

1 tsp salt

1/2 cup fresh parsley leaves, finely cut

black pepper, to taste

Directions:

Place the chicken, bay leaf, celery, carrot, onion, red pepper, sweet potato and salt into a pot with 5 cups of cold water.

Bring to the boil, reduce heat and simmer for 30 minutes. Season with salt and pepper, add in parsley, simmer for 2-3 minutes and serve.

Creamy Paleo Chicken Soup

Serves: 4

Prep time: 35 min

Ingredients:

4 chicken breasts

1 carrot, chopped

1 cup zucchini, peeled and chopped

2 cups cauliflower, broken into florets

1 celery rib, chopped

1 small onion, chopped

5 cups water

1/2 tsp salt

black pepper, to taste

Directions:

Place chicken breasts, onion, carrot, celery, cauliflower and zucchini in a deep soup pot. Add in salt, black pepper and 5 cups of water. Stir and bring to a boil.

Simmer for 30 minutes then remove chicken from the pot and let it cool slightly.

Blend soup until completely smooth. Shred or dice the chicken meat, return it back to the pot, stir and serve.

Broccoli and Chicken Soup

Serves: 4

Prep time: 35 min

Ingredients:

4 boneless chicken thighs, diced

1 small carrot, chopped

1 broccoli head, broken into florets

1 garlic clove, chopped

1 small onion, chopped

4 cups water

3 tbsp extra virgin olive oil

1/2 tsp salt

black pepper, to taste

Directions:

In a deep soup pot, heat olive oil and gently sauté broccoli for 2-3 minutes, stirring occasionally. Add in onion, carrot, chicken and cook, stirring, for 2-3 minutes. Stir in the salt, black pepper and water.

Bring to a boil. Simmer for 30 minutes then remove from heat and set aside to cool.

In a blender or food processor, blend soup until completely smooth. Serve and enjoy!

Walnut and Oregano Crusted Chicken

Serves: 4

Prep time: 35-40 min

Ingredients:

4 skinless, boneless chicken breasts

10-12 fresh oregano leaves

1/2 cup walnuts, chopped

2 garlic cloves, chopped

2 eggs, beaten

salt and pepper,to taste

Directions:

Blend the garlic, oregano and walnuts in a food processor until a rough crumb is formed. Season with salt and black pepper. Stir and place this mixture on a plate.

Whisk eggs in a deep bowl. Dip each chicken breast in the beaten egg then roll it in the walnut mixture. Place coated chicken on a baking tray and bake at 375 F for 13 minutes each side.

Walnut Pesto Stuffed Chicken

Serves: 4

Prep time: 35 min

Ingredients:

4 large chicken breasts

for the walnut pesto

1/2 cup walnuts, chopped

10 fresh basil leaves

1 garlic clove

1 tbsp chia seeds

2-3 green olives

4 tbsps extra virgin olive oil

1 tbsp lemon juice

salt and black pepper, to taste

Directions:

In a food processor, blend together walnuts, olives, basil, olive oil, garlic, chia seeds and lemon juice until completely smooth.

Carefully butterfly each chicken breast. Cover with plastic wrap and beat with a heavy object until the breast is flattened.

Put a tablespoon of the walnut mixture in each breast and roll over the top part like a flap. Season with salt and black pepper and bake at 375 F for 35 minutes.

Chicken with Olive Paste

Serves: 4

Prep time: 40 min

Ingredients:

2 chicken breasts (each cut into 2 cutlets)

2 garlic cloves, crushed

for the olive paste:

2 tbsp olive oil

2 cloves garlic, peeled

2/3 cup pitted black olives

2 tbsp capers

1 tbsp tomato paste

1 tbsp basil, chopped

3 tbsp extra virgin olive oil

Directions:

Place the garlic cloves into a food processor together with the olives, capers, basil, tomato paste and olive oil. Blend until smooth. Season to taste with salt and pepper.

Gently heat oil in a skillet on medium heat. Add in the chicken cutlets and cook each side for 4-5 minutes. Serve each cutlet topped with olive paste.

Chicken and Bacon Frittata

Serves: 4

Prep time: 35 min

Ingredients:

1/2 cup chicken, chopped finely

3 oz bacon, chopped

4-5 green onions, finely chopped

1 garlic clove, chopped

1 red bell pepper, diced

1 small tomato, diced

4 eggs whisked

4 tbsp coconut milk

1/2 tsp dried oregano

½ tsp dried parsley

4 tbsp extra virgin olive oil

salt, to taste

black pepper, to taste

Directions:

Heat two tablespoons of olive oil in a frying pan and gently cook the chicken until almost cooked through. Add the onions and garlic and cook for another minute. Set aside.

In the same pan, heat the remaining olive oil. Cook the bell pepper and tomato for 2-3 minutes, until lightly cooked. Add in the chicken, bacon and green onions, and mix well. Pour it all into a baking dish.

In a medium bowl, whisk eggs, coconut milk and seasonings together. Pour over the top of the meat and vegetable mixture, making sure that it covers it well. Bake in a preheated to 360 F oven for about 15 minutes, or until eggs are cooked through.

Chicken and Zucchini Frittata

Serves: 4

Prep time: 30 min

Ingredients:

1 cup chicken, chopped finely

1/2 onion, finely chopped

2 garlic cloves, chopped

1 zucchini, peeled and diced

1 tomato, diced

2 tbsp dill, finely chopped

4 eggs

3 tbsp coconut milk

4 tbsp olive oil

Directions:

Heat two tablespoons of olive oil in a frying pan and gently cook the chicken until almost cooked through. Add the onion and garlic and cook for another minute. Set aside.

In the same pan, heat the remaining olive oil. Cook the zucchini and tomato for for 3-4 minutes, until lightly cooked. Add in the chicken and mix everything well. Pour it all into the baking dish.

In a medium bowl, whisk eggs, coconut milk and dill together. Pour over the top of the chicken and vegetable mixture, making sure that it covers it well. Bake in a preheated to 360 F oven for around 15 minutes, until set. Garnish with fresh dill.

Hearty Chicken Spinach Frittata

Serves: 4

Prep time: 30 min

Ingredients:

1 cup chicken, chopped finely

3-4 green onions, finely chopped

5 oz frozen chopped spinach, defrosted and excess moisture squeezed out

½ zucchini, peeled and shredded

1 large tomato, thinly sliced

2 tbsp fresh rosemary leaves, finely chopped

5 eggs

3 tbsp coconut milk

4 tbsp olive oil

Directions:

Grease a shallow casserole dish. Heat two tablespoons of olive oil in a frying pan and gently cook the chicken until almost cooked through. Add in the onions and garlic and cook for another minute. Set aside.

In the same pan, heat the remaining olive oil. Cook the zucchini and spinach, stirring constantly, until lightly cooked. Add in the chicken mixture, and combine everything well. Pour it all into the casserole.

In a medium bowl, whisk eggs, coconut milk and rosemary together. Pour over the top of the chicken and vegetable mixture, making sure that it covers it well. Lay the tomato slices on top. Bake in a preheated to 360 F oven for around 15 minutes, until set. Garnish with rosemary.

Chicken and Mushroom Frittata

Serves: 4

Prep time: 20 min

Ingredients:

1 cup roasted chicken meat, chopped

1 cup white mushrooms, chopped

½ onion, chopped

2 garlic cloves, chopped

1 large tomato, thinly sliced

1/2 tsp salt

1/2 tsp black pepper

1 tsp dried thyme

4 large eggs, beaten well

2 tbsp extra virgin olive oil

Directions:

Grease a shallow casserole dish. Heat two tablespoons of olive oil in a frying pan and gently cook the onions and garlic until onion is transparent. Add in the mushrooms, stir, and cook on medium-high heat for 3-4 minutes. Add in the chicken and combine everything well. Pour it into the casserole.

In a medium bowl, whisk eggs, coconut milk, salt, black pepper and thyme together. Pour over the top of the chicken and mushroom mixture, making sure that it covers it well. Lay the tomato slices on top. Bake in a preheated to 360 F oven for around 15 minutes, until set.

Mediterranean Chicken Stew

Serves: 4

Prep time: 35 min

Ingredients:

4 chicken breasts

1 onion, chopped

1 small zucchini, peeled and chopped

1 red bell pepper, chopped

1 cup tomato sauce

1 cup assorted olives, pitted

1 tsp dried basil

1/2 cup fresh parsley, finely chopped

3 tbsp extra virgin olive oil

Directions:

In a deep pan, heat olive oil and seal the chicken breasts. Set aside in a plate.

In the same pan, gently sauté the onion and bell pepper, stirring, for 2-3 minutes, or until the onion has softened. Return chicken to the pan. Add in zucchini, tomato sauce, olives, basil, salt and pepper. Cover the pan and bring to a boil. Reduce heat and simmer for 30 minutes, or until the chicken is cooked through. Sprinkle with fresh parsley and serve.

Chicken and Onion Casserole

Serves: 4

Prep time: 35 min

Ingredients:

4 chicken breasts

4-5 large onions, sliced

2 leeks, cut

1 cup black olives, pitted

4 tbsp extra virgin olive oil

1 tsp thyme

salt and black pepper, to taste

Directions:

Heat olive oil in a large, deep frying pan over medium-high heat. Brown chicken, turning, for 2-3 minutes each side or until golden. Set aside in a casserole dish.

Cut the onions and leeks and add them on and around the chicken, Add in olives, thyme, salt and black pepper to taste. Cover with a lid or aluminum foil and bake at 375 F for 35 minutes, or until the chicken is cooked through. Uncover and return to the oven for 5 minutes or until chicken is crispy.

Chicken and Mushrooms

Serves: 4

Prep time: 20-30 min

Ingredients:

4 chicken breasts, diced

2 lbs mushrooms, chopped

1 onion, chopped

4 tbsp extra virgin olive oil

1 tbsp thyme

1 tbsp lemon rind

salt and black, pepper to taste

Directions:

Heat olive oil in a deep frying pan over medium-high heat. Brown chicken, stirring, for 2 minutes each side, or until golden.

Add the chopped onion, mushrooms, lemon rind, salt and black pepper, and stir to combine.

Reduce heat, cover and simmer for 30 minutes. Uncover and simmer for 5 more minutes.

Chicken Drumstick Casserole

Serves: 4

Prep time: 35 min

Ingredients:

8 chicken drumsticks

1 head broccoli, cut into florets

1 leek, sliced

1 garlic clove, crushed

1 sweet potato, peeled and cubed

1 carrot, cut

1 tsp dried rosemary

4 tbsp olive oil

1 tsp dried oregano

salt and black pepper, to taste

Directions:

Heat the olive oil in a non stick frying pan over medium heat. Add the chicken drumsticks and cook, turning occasionally, for 3-4 minutes, or until sealed.

Transfer chicken to a casserole and add in the vegetables. Sprinkle with salt, pepper and oregano and bake in a preheated to 375 F oven until cooked through.

Hunter Style Chicken

Serves: 4

Prep time: 45 min

Ingredients:

1 chicken (3-4 lbs), cut into pieces

1 onions, sliced

2 red peppers, sliced

6-7 white mushrooms, sliced

1 can tomatoes, diced and drained

3 garlic cloves, thinly sliced

2 tbsp extra virgin olive oil

salt and black pepper, to taste

1/2 cup parsley leaves, finely cut

Directions:

Heat olive oil in a deep pan on medium heat. Working in batches, brown the chicken pieces, for 5-6 minutes each side. Add in the onions, garlic and peppers together with the mushrooms and canned tomatoes.

Lower the heat and cover the pan with the lid slightly ajar.

Let the chicken simmer for about 40 minutes, turning from time to time. Sprinkle with parsley, set aside to rest a few minutes before serving to keep the juices inside and serve.

Healthy Chicken Meatballs

Serves: 4-5

Prep time: 30 min

Ingredients:

2 lbs ground chicken meat

1 onion, very finely cut

2 eggs, lightly whisked

1 tbsp chia seeds

1 tbsp parsley, finely chopped

1 tbs ground ginger

1/2 tsp cumin

2 tbsp extra virgin olive oil

1 cup chicken broth

1 can tomatoes, drained and diced

1 tbsp tomato paste

Directions:

Preheat the oven to 350 F. Line a baking tray with baking paper.

Combine the ground chicken, onion, eggs, chia seeds, parsley, ginger, salt and cumin in a bowl. Using your hands, mix until everything until it is combined well. Roll chicken mixture into walnut sized meatballs and arrange them on the baking tray. Bake for 10 minutes until light golden.

In a deep frying pan, heat olive oil medium heat. Stir in remaining ginger. Add in tomatoes and stir. Add chicken broth and tomato paste, and bring to a boil, then reduce heat and simmer for 5 minutes. Add the meatballs and simmer for 20 more minutes or until the meat is cooked through and the sauce has thickened.

Bacon Wrapped Chicken Breasts

Serves: 4

Prep time: 45 min

Ingredients:

2 large boneless chicken breasts

10 slices sugar-free bacon

3-4 canned artichoke hearts, chopped

3-4 sun-dried tomatoes, finely chopped

2 garlic cloves, crushed

a few fresh rosemary leaves, chopped

Mix the artichoke hearts and the sun-dried tomatoes in a small bowl.

Directions:

Preheat the oven to 375 F. Carefully butterfly each chicken breast ensuring not to slice all the way through. Season with salt and spoon ¼ of the stuffing in the middle of each breast. Spread it as evenly as possible and roll the breasts tightly. Wrap two slices of bacon around each chicken breast and secure the bacon with a toothpick.

Arrange the chicken rolls in a baking dish, cover with a lid or aluminum foil and bake at 375 F for 35 minutes. Remove foil and return to the oven for 10 minutes or until bacon is crispy.

Sun-dried Tomatoes Stuffed Chicken Breasts

Serves: 4

Prep time: 35-40 min

Ingredients:

4 boneless, skinless chicken breasts

8 slices sugar-free bacon

12 sun dried tomatoes

4 tbsp chopped black olives

4 tbsp tahini

salt and pepper, to taste

Directions:

Preheat oven to 375 Degrees F. Carefully butterfly open the chicken breasts but do not slice all the way through. Season with salt and pepper and spread one tablespoon tahini all over the inside of each breast.

Add in three sun-dried tomatoes, a tablespoon of olives, and fold the chicken breasts closed back onto itself. Wrap two slices of bacon around each chicken breast and secure the bacon with a toothpick.

Arrange the chicken rolls in a baking dish, cover with aluminum foil and bake at 375 F for 35 minutes. Remove foil and return to the oven for 10 minutes or until bacon is crispy.

Spicy Chicken Strips

Serves: 4

Prep time: 40 min

Ingredients:

3 boneless, skinless chicken breasts, cut into strips

1/4 cup white wine

1 tsp paprika

1 tsp dried oregano

1 tbsp garlic powder

1 tsp tumeric

½ tsp chili powder

Directions:

Cut each chicken breast into 4-5 small strips. Place the strips in a large bowl and add the wine and spices. Stir, so the spices distribute evenly and place in the fridge for about 20 minutes.

Line a large baking tray and arrange the chicken pieces. Bake in a preheated to 350 F oven for about 20 minutes or until done.

Healthy Chicken Dippers

Serves: 4

Prep time: 20 min

Ingredients:

1 pound boneless, skinless chicken breast, cut into thin strips

2 egg, whisked

1/2 cup shredded coconut

1/4 cup almond flour

1 tbsp sesame seeds

1 tsp garlic powder

1/3 tsp salt

2 tbsp extra virgin olive oil

Directions:

Preheat oven to 350 F. Whisk the eggs in a small bowl. In another bowl, mix the coconut, almond flour, sesame seeds, garlic powder and salt. Dip each chicken strip in the whisked eggs, then in the coconut mixture. Coat on all sides and set aside on a plate.

Place a large skillet over medium heat. Add olive oil and when it is hot add in some of the strips. Cook for about two minutes then flip each chicken strip and cook on the other side. Set aside to cool and serve.

Spicy Mustard Chicken

Serves: 4

Prep time: 65 min

Ingredients:

4 chicken breasts

2 garlic cloves, crushed

1/2 cup chicken broth

3 tbsp Dijon mustard

2 tbsp extra virgin olive oil

1 tsp chili powder

Directions:

In a small bowl, mix mustard, olive oil, chicken broth, garlic and chili. Marinate the chicken for 30 minutes. Bake at 375 F for 35 minutes.

Garlic Chicken

Serves: 4

Prep time: 35 min

Ingredients:

4 boneless skinless chicken breasts

5 garlic cloves, crushed

3 lemon slices

6-7 green olives, pitted

1 tbsp dried rosemary

2 tbsp extra virgin olive oil

salt and pepper, to taste

Directions:

Gently heat the olive oil in a skillet over medium-low heat and sauté the garlic for about a minute, stirring.

Add the lemon slices to the bottom of the pan. Lay the chicken breasts on top of the lemon. Add in the rosemary and the olives. Season with salt and pepper to taste, cover the pan, and cook, on medium-low, for 20 minutes or until the chicken breasts are cooked through, turning once. Uncover and cook for 2-3 minutes, until the liquid evaporates.

Chicken Puttanesca

Serves: 4

Prep time: 30 min

Ingredients:

4 boneless chicken breasts

2 tbsp extra virgin olive oil

for the sauce:

2 tbsp extra virgin olive oil

4 garlic cloves, crushed

1 small onion, diced

1/2 cup green olives, pitted and chopped

2 tbsp capers, drained and coarsely chopped

3 boneless anchovy filets, coarsely chopped

2 tomatoes, diced

1 tbsp tomato paste

1/2 tsp paprika

salt and black pepper, to taste

Directions:

Heat two tablespoons of olive oil in a large skillet and brown the chicken for about 2 minutes, each side. Cover with a lid and cook for about 10-15 minutes, or until cooked through. Set aside on 4 plates.

In the same skillet, heat two tablespoons of olive oil. Add in garlic, onions, anchovies, olives, capers and paprika. Gently sauté these ingredients, stirring constantly, for about one minute.

Add in the tomatoes and tomato paste, season with salt and pepper and cook over high heat for 5-6 minutes or until the tomatoes are cooked and the sauce thickens.

Divide the sauce between the chicken breasts and serve.

Grilled Chicken with Herbs

Serves: 4

Prep time: 50 min

Ingredients:

8 chicken thigh or 4 chicken breasts

½ cup parsley leaves

¼ cup oregano leaves

¼ cup cilantro leaves

3 garlic cloves, crushed

2 tbsp extra virgin olive oil

½ tsp salt

1/2 tsp tumeric

Directions:

Place the garlic, herbs, olive oil, salt, paprika and tumeric in a food processor or blender and pulse until smooth. Pour this mixture over the chicken and stir to coat meat well. Refrigerate for at least 20 minutes.

Arrange the chicken on a baking tray and bake for 30 minutes or until cooked through.

Greek Style Chicken Skewers

Serves: 4

Prep time: 50 min

Ingredients:

2 lbs chicken breasts, diced

4 small zucchinis, diced

3 tbsp extra virgin olive oil

1 lemon, juiced

2 garlic cloves, crushed

1 tsp dried oregano

1 tsp dried rosemary

12 wooden skewers

Directions:

Thread chicken and zucchini alternately onto each of 12 skewers. Place in a shallow dish. Combine extra virgin olive oil and lemon juice, garlic and oregano.

Pour over chicken. Turn to coat. Marinate for at least 30 minutes.

Preheat a barbecue plate on medium-high heat. Cook skewers for 4 minutes each side or until chicken is just cooked through.

Moroccan Paleo Chicken

Serves: 4

Prep time: 50 min

Ingredients:

1 whole chicken (3-4 lbs), cut into pieces

1 large onion, chopped

3 garlic cloves, chopped

1 tsp ginger

1 tsp cumin

1 tsp tumeric

salt and black pepper, to taste

1/2 cup assorted olives, pitted

1 preserved lemon, quartered

4 tbsp extra virgin olive oil

a bunch of fresh parsley

Directions:

In a deep bowl, mix three tablespoons of olive oil, onion, garlic, salt, ginger, cumin and tumeric. Combine these ingredients very well.

Add the chicken pieces into this mixture and set aside for 15 minutes.

Heat a baking dish on medium heat and add two tablespoons of olive oil. Add in the chicken and pour the remaining marinade over the top. Add olives and the preserved lemon.

Tie the parsley and place on top of the chicken. Cover with a lid or aluminum foil and bake in a preheated to 375 F oven for 45 minutes or until the chicken is cooked through.

Remove the parsley and serve.

Chicken with Almonds and Prunes

Serves: 4

Prep time: 20 min

Ingredients:

2 lb boneless chicken thighs, trimmed

1 cup fresh orange juice

1/2 cup pitted prunes

1/4 cup blanched almonds

3 tbsp raisins

1 tsp ground cinnamon

1 tsp tumeric

salt and black pepper, to taste

1/4 cup parsley, chopped

Directions:

In a deep pan, combine orange juice with prunes, almonds, raisins and cinnamon.

Bring to a boil then reduce heat to medium-low and boil for 5-6 minutes or until liquid is reduced by half.

Add in the chicken, cover and simmer for 15 minutes or until cooked through. Season to taste with salt and pepper, sprinkle with parsley and serve.

Paleo Moussaka

Serves: 6

Prep time: 45 min

Ingredients:

2 eggplants, peeled and cut into thick rounds

1 tbsp salt

1 large onion, chopped

2 garlic cloves, crushed

1/2 tsp ground cinnamon

1/2 tsp ground nutmeg

1/4 tsp ground coriander

1/4 tsp ground ginger

1 can tomatoes, undrained, chopped

3 cups cooked chicken, shredded

1/2 cup parsley leaves, finely chopped

2 eggs

3 tbsp coconut milk

4 tbsp extra virgin olive oil

salt and black pepper, to taste

Directions:

Peel and cut the eggplant and place the slices on a plate. Sprinkle with a tablespoon of salt and set aside for 30 minutes, then rinse and pat dry.

Heat olive oil in a deep frying pan over medium-high heat. Fry the eggplant slices in batches for 2-3 minutes each side or until golden. Set aside in a plate.

In the same pan, sauté onion and garlic for 2-3 minutes or until transparent. Add spice and sauté for one minute then add in tomatoes. Simmer until the tomato sauce thickness. Add shredded chicken, parsley and stir to combine.

Place half the eggplant slices in an ovenproof baking dish. Cover with chicken and tomato mixture and top with remaining eggplant.

Whisk two eggs with coconut milk. Pour over the meat and eggplant mixture. Bake for 30 minutes or until golden. Set aside for five minutes and serve.

Easy Chicken and Broccoli Stir-fry

Serves: 6

Prep time: 35 min

Ingredients:

4 chicken breasts, cut in strips

1 small red onion, thinly sliced

3 garlic cloves, chopped

1 head broccoli, cut into small florets

1/2 cup raw cashew nuts

3 tbsp virgin coconut oil

1 tsp ginger powder

1/2 tsp coriander

salt and black pepper, to taste

Directions:

Combine the shredded coconut with salt and black pepper and coat well all chicken pieces.

Heat oil in a large non-stick frying pan and cook the chicken until golden. Add the ginger, coriander, red onion and garlic and stir-fry for another minute. Add in the broccoli and cashews and stir fry until cooked to your liking.

FREE BONUS RECIPES: 20 Superfood Paleo and Vegan Smoothies for Vibrant Health and Easy Weight Loss

Kale and Kiwi Smoothie

Serves: 2

Prep time: 2-3 min

Ingredients:

2-3 ice cubes

1 cup orange juice

1 small pear, peeled and chopped

2 kiwi, peeled and chopped

2-3 kale leaves

2-3 dates, pitted

Directions:

Combine all ingredients in a high speed blender and blend until smooth.

Delicious Broccoli Smoothie

Serves: 2

Prep time: 2-3 min

Ingredients:

2-3 frozen broccoli florets

1 cup coconut milk

1 banana, peeled and chopped

1 cup pineapple, cut

1 peach, chopped

1 tsp cinnamon

Directions:

Combine all ingredients in a high speed blender and blend until smooth.

Papaya Smoothie

Serves: 2

Prep time: 2-3 min

Ingredients:

2-3 frozen broccoli florets

1 cup orange juice

1 small ripe avocado, peeled, cored and diced

1 cup papaya

1 cup fresh strawberries

Directions:

Combine all ingredients in a high speed blender and blend until smooth.

Beet and Papaya Smoothie

Serves: 2

Prep time: 2-3 min

Ingredients:

3-4 ice cubes

1 cup orange juice

1 banana, peeled and chopped

1 cup papaya

1 small beet, peeled and cut

Directions:

Combine all ingredients in a high speed blender and blend until smooth.

Lean Green Smoothie

Serves: 2

Prep time: 2-3 min

Ingredients:

1 frozen banana, chopped

1 cup orange juice

2-3 kale leaves, stems removed

1 small cucumber, peeled and chopped

1/2 cup fresh parsley leaves

½ tsp grated ginger

Directions:

Combine all ingredients in a high speed blender and blend until smooth.

Easy Antioxidant Smoothie

Serves: 2

Prep time: 2-3 min

Ingredients:

2-3 frozen broccoli florets

1 cup orange juice

2 plums, cut

1 cup raspberries

1 tsp ginger powder

Directions:

Combine all ingredients in a high speed blender and blend until smooth.

Healthy Purple Smoothie

Serves: 2

Prep time: 2-3 min

Ingredients:

2-3 frozen broccoli florets

1 cup water

1/2 avocado, peeled and chopped

3 plums, chopped

1 cup blueberries

Directions:

Combine all ingredients in a high speed blender and blend until smooth.

Mom's Favorite Kale Smoothie

Serves: 2

Prep time: 2-3 min

Ingredients:

2-3 ice cubes

1½ cup orange juice

1 green small apple, cut

½ cucumber, chopped

2-3 leaves kale

½ cup raspberries

Directions:

Combine all ingredients in a high speed blender and blend until smooth.

Creamy Green Smoothie

Serves: 2

Prep time: 2-3 min

Ingredients:

1 frozen banana

1 cup coconut milk

1 small pear, chopped

1 cup baby spinach

1 cup grapes

1 tbsp coconut butter

1 tsp vanilla extract

Directions:

Combine all ingredients in a high speed blender and blend until smooth.

Strawberry and Arugula Smoothie

Serves: 2

Prep time: 2-3 min

Ingredients:

2 cups frozen strawberries

1 cup unsweetened almond milk

10-12 arugula leaves

1/2 tsp ground cinnamon

Directions:

Combine ice, almond milk, strawberries, arugula and cinnamon in a high speed blender. Blend until smooth and serve.

Emma's Amazing Smoothie

Serves: 2

Prep time: 2-3 min

Ingredients:

1 frozen banana, chopped

1 cup orange juice

1 large nectarine, sliced

1/2 zucchini, peeled and chopped

2-3 dates, pitted

Directions:

Combine all ingredients in a high speed blender and blend until smooth.

Good-To-Go Morning Smoothie

Serves: 2

Prep time: 2-3 min

Ingredients:

1 cup frozen strawberries

1 cup apple juice

1 banana, chopped

1 cup raw asparagus, chopped

1 tbsp ground flaxseed

Directions:

Combine all ingredients in a high speed blender and blend until smooth.

Endless Energy Smoothie

Serves: 2

Prep time: 2-3 min

Ingredients:

1 frozen banana, chopped

11/2 cup green tea

1 cup chopped pineapple

2 raw asparagus spears, chopped

1 lime, juiced

1 tbsp chia seeds

Directions:

Combine all ingredients in a high speed blender and blend until smooth.

High-fibre Fruit Smoothie

Serves: 2

Prep time: 2-3 min

Ingredients:

1 frozen banana, chopped

1 cup orange juice

2 cups chopped papaya

1 cup shredded cabbage

1 tbsp chia seeds

Directions:

Combine all ingredients in a high speed blender and blend until smooth.

Nutritious Green Smoothie

Serves: 2

Prep time: 2-3 min

Ingredients:

2-3 frozen broccoli florets

1 cup apple juice

1 large pear, chopped

1 kiwi, peeled and chopped

1 cup spinach leaves

1-2 dates, pitted

Directions:

Combine all ingredients in a high speed blender and blend until smooth.

Apricot, Strawberry and Banana Smoothie

Serves: 2

Prep time: 2-3 min

Ingredients:

1 frozen banana

11/2 cup almond milk

5 dried apricots

1 cup fresh strawberries

Directions:

Combine all ingredients in a high speed blender and blend until smooth.

Spinach and Green Apple Smoothie

Serves: 2

Prep time: 2-3 min

Ingredients:

3-4 ice cubes

1 cup unsweetened almond milk

1 banana, peeled and chopped

2 green apples, peeled and chopped

1 cup raw spinach leaves

3-4 dates, pitted

1 tsp grated ginger

Directions:

Combine all ingredients in a high speed blender and blend until smooth.

Superfood Blueberry Smoothie

Serves: 2

Prep time: 2-3 min

Ingredients:

2-3 cubes frozen spinach

1 cup green tea

1 banana

2 cups blueberries

1 tbsp ground flaxseed

Directions:

Combine all ingredients in a high speed blender and blend until smooth.

Zucchini and Blueberry Smoothie

Serves: 2

Prep time: 2-3 min

Ingredients:

1 cup frozen blueberries

1 cup unsweetened almond milk

1 banana

1 zucchini, peeled and chopped

Directions:

Combine all ingredients in a high speed blender and blend until smooth.

Tropical Spinach Smoothie

Serves: 2

Prep time: 2-3 min

Ingredients:

1/2 cup crushed ice or 3-4 ice cubes

1 cup coconut milk

1 mango, peeled and diced

1 cup fresh spinach leaves

4-5 dates, pitted

1/2 tsp vanilla extract

Directions:

Combine all ingredients in a high speed blender and blend until smooth.

About the Author

Alissa Grey lives in a small French village in the foothills of a beautiful mountain range with her husband, three teenage kids, two free spirited dogs, and various other animals.

She is incredibly lucky to be able to cook and eat natural foods, mostly grown nearby, something she's done since she was a teenager. Alissa enjoys reading, hanging out with her family, going for long hikes, and growing organic vegetables and herbs.

80190498R00052

Made in the USA
Columbia, SC
04 November 2017